# Walk-a-thon: The Ultimate Guide to Walking a Half Marathon or Marathon Race!

by Scott O. Morton

LERK Publishing, LLC

Cover design: LERK Publishing, LLC

ISBN: **978-1-947010-29-1** (Paperback)

# Follow me:

Facebook: facebook.com/BeginnerToFinisher

SoundCloud: https://soundcloud.com/scott-morton-231690676

Twitter: https://twitter.com/BeginR2FinishR

Instagram: https://www.instagram.com/beginner2finisher/

Tumblr: https://beginnertofinisherrunning.tumblr.com/

Website: www.halfmarathonforbeginners.com

Email: scottmorton@halfmarathonforbeginners.com

To my sisters, Gayla and Cristie

## Table of Contents

# Medical Disclaimer

The information in this book is meant to supplement, not replace, proper half marathon training. A sport involving speed, equipment, balance and environmental factors, and running, will involve some inherent risk. The authors and publisher advise readers to take full responsibility for their safety and know their limits. Before practicing the skills described in this book, be sure that your equipment is well maintained, and do not take risks beyond your level of experience, aptitude, training, and comfort level.

If you have sports related injuries, I highly suggest that you talk to a medical professional to determine if you are fit enough to endure running. Not seeking medical advice could further exacerbate an existing injury. I am not a legal or medical professional, nor am I offering any type of legal or medical advice. One last time, if you're injured or have medical conditions that prevent you from taking on a rigorous running training program, please seek the opinion of a licensed physician before participating in any physical training. While the training required for a half marathon is not nearly as difficult as the training for a full marathon, it will still push both your mental and physical capabilities.

# Other Books by Scott O. Morton

## Beginner to Finisher Series:

**Book 1:** _Why New Runners Fail: 26 Ultimate Tips You Should Know Before You Start Running!_

**Book 2**: _5K Fury: 10 Proven Steps to Get You to the Finish Line in 9 weeks or less!_

**Book 3:** _10K Titan: Push Beyond the 5K in 6 Weeks or Less!_

**Book 4:** _Beginner's Guide to Half Marathons: A Simple Step-By-Step Solution to Get You to the Finish Line in 12 Weeks!_

**Book 5:** _Long Run Hacks: 20 Ultimate Tips to Help You Push Through Hard Runs!_

**Book 6:** _How to Avoid a Half Marathon Meltdown: 10 Things You Need to Know to Make Sure Your First Half Marathon Isn't Your Last!_

**Book 7:** _Marathon Machine - Breakthrough Your Running Barrier in 18 weeks and Conquer Your Dream! (COMING SOON)_

## FREE to read with a Kindle Unlimited Subscription (below only):

*Beginner's Guide to Half Marathons: 12 Week Training Workbook*

## Supercharge Your Walking Life Series:

**Book 1:** *42,000 Steps: 100 simple ways to maximize your daily step count!*

**Book 2:** *Supercharged Walking: 20 Simple Methods to Help You Level Up Your Stride!*

**Book 3:** *Walk-a-thon - The Ultimate Guide to Walking a Half Marathon or Marathon Race!*

**Book 4:** *Walk yourself to a healthier fitter you, by discovering meditation walking: 20 easy steps to jump start your meditating!*

# Why I Wrote This Book

I wrote this book for walkers with the desire to push beyond the 5K. If no serious medical conditions lie in your way, everyone should be able to walk at least a half marathon. Will it be extremely easy? The answer is found in how good of shape you are in. The 5K, commonly known as the gateway race, is by far the most the most popular race. The 10K would be the next steps in line for walking your way to a half marathon and a full marathon. If you follow the training and steps outlined in this book, you can complete these races.

# What's in This Book?

This book will cover the essentials of walking a half marathon or marathon race. While the half marathon is completely doable, the marathon is a little trickier to tackle. This book will take you through walking the longer duration races such as the half marathon and the marathon.

This book DOES NOT cover walking a 5K or 10K. If you need to start at the 5K or 10K race please see my other books section (two pages back) and read *5K Fury* or *10K Titan*. These two books are for runners but can easily be walked as well.

### Birds eye view of the book:

**Part I** - Essentials of walking: will take you through proper form of a walk, the differences between running and walking, as well as walking gear and attire.

**Part II** - Pre-training requirements for a half marathon and marathon race.

**Part III** - The half marathon: this section will focus on walking the half marathon and essentials needed to know to finish within the cutoff time.

**Part IV** - The marathon: this is the trickiest of all to finish by just walking. I will dive into a few strategies that could help you finish the marathon by walking before your time runs out.

**Part V** - This section provides essential go to information on days leading up to race day followed by post-race activities.

# Assumptions

Before you dive into this book, I'm assuming the following:

- You can walk at least a couple of miles a day.
- You will stick to a training schedule that is provided in this book or elsewhere.
- You have a desire to walk the much bigger and longer races.
- You want to walk a half or full marathon.

If you are having trouble completing a 1-2-mile walk, I suggest trying to get to the point where you can walk at least two miles before continuing with this book. If weight is an issue or your joints are under too much stress to be able to walk a few miles, I would investigate walking in the water. When you walk in the water you are putting far less stress on your joints and bones and able to walk greater distances. Yes, it is somewhat slower to walk in water, but you can get up to speed quickly if you use this approach.

# Part I - Essentials of Walking

# Race - Bare Bones What You Need to Know

## *Research the Race before you Pace*

You are super excited! You've finally comes to terms that you can walk a half marathon and/or a marathon race. Stop right there! I'm not going to burst your bubble. I just want you to be sure you know which race you are getting yourself and your feet into. Many races say they are walker friendly but turn out to not be so walker friendly in the end. Please don't think I'm being a negative Nick, I'm silently routing for all walkers who can tackle the big races. Here is a list of things that commonly go wrong in a "walker friendly" race:

- The race ends before the cut off time.
- The race ends and all race course road help has been abandoned and full road rules are back in effect.
- You cross the finish line and all the medals are gone (yes this happens!).
- You cross the finish line and all the food has been eaten.
- You cross the finish line and all medical volunteer help has vacated the course.
- You're unable to keep a pace (normally greater than 15 minutes/mile), and they flag you down and require you to ride in a vehicle to the finish line (yes this happens, especially at the Disney races!)

# Important Pre-Race Tip

Can you guess what the number one most important pre-race factor is for race participants that plan on walking longer races? It's not the ability to walk a half marathon or marathon, although this would be number two on my list. I'll give you a hint. The answer has to do with time.

The number one most important pre-race factor is, the course cutoff time. Why is the course cut off time the most important pre-race factor?

Here is a list of the three most important pre-race factors for participants planning on walking a long duration race:
   1) Know the cutoff time.
   2) Do you have the physical ability to walk the full duration of the race?
   3) Is the race "walker" friendly?

# Cutoff Time

One might argue that you need to know whether you have the physical ability to walk a race. I do agree with this argument; however, I believe that you need to know the race course limits before you can make the decision whether or not you can sustain walking the duration of the race within the cutoff window.

# Physical Ability

If you know the course cut off time you can estimate whether you will be physically able to cross the finish line within the time constraints of the course. For most walkers, having the physical ability to finish a 5K, 10K, or 15K is simple and straight forward. This is easy to accomplish because you are only on your feet for a maximum of about 3 hours in the case of a 15K (9.3 miles). After 3 hours, especially in running, everything starts plummeting to the ground. Your energy levels drop causing your mental ability to focus to come under attack by negative thoughts. This in turn slows you down and starts to eat away at your mental and physical ability to finish a race.

# Walker Friendly

When a race is considered "Walker Friendly," that normally means that the race caters to both the runner and walker. However, and that's a big however, most longer duration races that are simply "Walker Friendly" doesn't

necessarily mean that they're completely "Walker Friendly." Some races, even though they claim they are "Walker Friendly," they still require walkers to keep a particular pace and finish within a time window. Most half marathons have strict cut off times of 4 hours. While, most marathons have a strict cut off time of 7 hours (some of them 6 hours or less). The best way to determine the level of a "Walker Friendly" race, is to research and contact a specific half Marathon or marathon race director. Remember that most races, especially the 5K or 10K, can easily be finished at a casual walk pace. The races that you must pay closer attention to are the 15K and above.

## Walker Etiquette for Races

I have included this section for newer walkers, that have participated in shorter distances. If you follow these simple walker rules you should get along with everyone just fine on race day. Some of the tips are just common sense, while others you will find valuable.

Etiquette for Walkers:

1) Start in the correct corral. If you're walking the race, you're going to be in the last corral. If your race doesn't have corrals, then position yourself at the very back of the herd of people when lining up to start.
2) Stay to the right of the course so people can pass you on the left.

3) Know the race cutoff time and know your pace so that you can finish on time.
4) Don't stop at the water station and block traffic, grab a water and keep walking.
5) If there is a national anthem, out of respect, please stop talking until it's over.
6) Don't walk with more than 2 people abreast (side by side). When you get 3 or 4 walkers stacked up shoulder to shoulder, it tends to form a walking wall.
7) If you're going to take mid-race photos please be aware of other racers and move to the side to snap that photo.

## Walker Only Races

Your best bet is to find a long-distance race that is for walkers only. One walker only race that is popular in the United States, is called the Boston Marathon Jimmy Fund Walk. Running is not allowed for safety reasons. The course is open for at least 8 hours if not a little longer. If you live in the U.S.A. and you want to walk a marathon, here is a perfect location for you to get the job done. Plus, the cause is a great one. Dana-Farber Cancer Institute uses the fund to help fight cancer in young children. The race is towards the end of the month every year in September.

# Walking Form

## *Arms*

Sit on the ground and practice swinging your arms. Your hands should never touch the ground.

Arms bent at the waist level and swing them as you walk.

## *Body*

You don't need to lean forward like running. Just stand straight up and walk like you normally would.

## *Legs*

Don't over stride, this will make you more tired. Try for short strides with smaller steps.

## *Troubleshooting*

The bottom line is that walking should be natural. If your walking form doesn't seem natural or something hurts, then something is obliviously wrong. Walking should never hurt. On the other hand, running, can hurt from time to time when you are trying to work out some kinks in your muscles.

# Walking vs. Running

## *Two main factors*

Two main factors that underscore the differences between walking and running are intensity and impact. Your muscles are being used at a much more intense rate when you run versus when you walk. The impact of hitting the ground is much higher during running than when walking. The muscles that are used are the same, however, a person who runs versus a person who walks will be able to tone the muscles much quicker.

The main difference between walking and jogging is how the foot muscles work. When you're jogging, the ankle plantar flexors and knee extensors propel you. Walking, by comparison, uses the knee and hip extensors along with the plantar flexors – the deep muscles in your lower leg.

Walking, for instance, may improve your balance and coordination, build core strength and lower your risk of developing heart disease, diabetes and high blood pressure. Plus, it aids in weight management and lifts your mood.

Over time, your muscles become more efficient at utilizing fat and oxygen for exercise, leading to improved physical performance.

# Advantages

Walking does have some advantages over running. Here are a few advantages that walkers have:

- Your energy doesn't get depleted as quickly.
- No need for extensive, strenuous training to build up your energy stores.
- The pictures that you take aren't nearly as blurry.
- Might meet new people that you can talk to along the race course.
- You won't sweat as much so you probably don't need as much water/Gatorade as a runner
- Able to eat more wholesome foods. When you run the food jostles quite a bit in your stomach. Walking doesn't make your body shift around as much as running making the food stay put. You might even stop for a slice of pizza!

# Disadvantages

Some disadvantages of walking are:

- You will be on your feet longer, so you need to make sure you can walk the full distance required.
- Your cutoff time becomes more critical in longer races such as the half marathon or marathon.
- You will need more fuel due to exercising for a longer period.
- You might not finish the race if you don't keep up your pace.
- All the post-race food might be gone by the time you're finished.
- You might not get a medal if they run out.
- You might get a race status of "DNF" which stands for "Did Not Finish," if you get picked up by the pace police.

# *Part II - Pre-Training Requirements*

# Pre-training Assessment

Before you start your training for your half or full marathon there are a few things you need to determine for yourself:

- How many consecutive miles can you walk without being exhausted?
- At what pace can you walk the above-mentioned miles without being exhausted?
- How long do you have to train before the race?
- What is your race day goal?
- Do you have any injuries that can prevent you from walking the full race?

# How far can you walk and at what pace?

Let's divide you into two different groups. The first group is for active walkers. People that walk between 3 and 5 miles at least 4 times a week. The second group is for walkers that occasionally go walking maybe once or twice a week. You walk a couple of miles and you're done.

For the people that are in the active walkers group you should be able to walk for 5+ miles easily 3+ times a week and not feel exhausted after walking 5 miles. The second group of walkers are the walkers that don't walk habitually 4+ times a week. If you tried to walk 5 miles three days in a row your body would more than likely feel tired.

Walking assessment:

Before you start training you need to assess where you're at when it comes to your walking fitness level. You can do this using a tread mill or a GPS watch or smart phone and an outdoor location (i.e. a track or park). I highly recommend an outdoor park where you have a loop location such as your car to keep liquids and snacks handy for your assessment. For most walkers your average pace will probably fall between 17 and 20 minutes per mile (10:33 and 12:26 minutes per kilometer). Can you walk faster than this? Yes. Some walkers walk almost as fast as the slowest runners.

For this assessment you need to be able to walk at or under 20 minutes a mile (12:26 minutes per kilometer). Walking faster than 20 minutes a mile is OK. Why should you not keep a pace greater than 20 minutes per mile? If you keep a pace that is greater than 20 minutes a mile (12:26 minutes per km), you run the risk of not completing the race before the cutoff time.

Walk for 5 miles and assess how you feel. If you feel OK and not exhausted, then go ahead and start pushing yourself an additional mile. Remember we are looking for a tired state and your legs might be a tiny bit sore. If you walk the 6th miles and you still feel OK and not winded push another mile. Keep repeating until you reach 10 miles, or your body becomes tired and you feel like you could still walk a few more miles. This is the point you want to stop at. Also, remember that when you're training, you need to drink fluids and snack if you feel hungry. The total number of miles you walked during your assessment will be able to tell you what weeks you can skip when you begin your training.

Let's say you walked 10 miles and felt more and more tired but not exhausted. Your breathing was controlled, and your legs might be a little sore. Since you completed 10 miles, you can , skip ahead on the half marathon training schedule or marathon schedule. What I typically do is subtract 1 mile from the total miles walked during the assessment. In this case, 10 miles walked - 1 mile is equal to 9 miles. Locate the long duration run on the training schedule which is 9 in this example. This is the location on the schedule where you can start your half marathon training.

In this case, you would be able to start at week number 6 or 7 for the half marathon race. For the marathon this would be week number 4. For kilometers, using the above example, it would be 14.4 kilometers (9 miles) which would be the same location on the training schedule for kilometers.

## What is your race day goal?

Your race day goal is the most important part of your training and race. As I've already stated in the previous chapters, walking requires a little different strategy than running. You really have three different strategies when you're walking a half marathon or marathon race. These three strategies are trying to finish the race before the race cutoff time, trying to finish at a defined time (your goal time), Trying to finish the race regardless of time (even beyond the race cutoff time).

You are trying to finish the race just before the cutoff time. The easiest way to accomplish this is determine which race you are going to walk. If you're walking a half marathon, most half marathons have a strict cutoff time of 4 hours. If you're walking a marathon most marathons have a strict cutoff time of 6 or 7 hours. If you're planning on walking a half marathon and you're a slow-paced walker your best choice for a half marathon would be a race that is on the same course as a marathon. This will turn your cutoff time into 6 or 7 hours for a half marathon race. With 6 or 7 hours available to complete the race most walkers should have no problem completing the race. The marathon is a lot trickier.

I created pacing tables to show you the total time it takes to finish a race at a certain pace. These are located at the end of the chapter.

**Example 1:**

If you walk at an extremely casual pace of 20 minutes per mile (12:26 minutes per km) you would finish a half

marathon in 4 hours and 22 minutes and a marathon in 8 hours and 44 minutes.

**Example 2:**

If you walk at a faster pace of 16 minutes per mile (9:58 minutes per km) you would finish a half marathon in 3 hours and 30 minutes and a marathon in 7 hours.

The second strategy would be to finish the race at your own defined total race time. In order to do this, you can look at the pacing tables below and determine your finish times and see what your pace needs to be. Let me point out that when you drop below 15 minutes per mile, some type of running will more than likely be involved. Walking at a pace of 15 minutes a mile can be done, but it's an extremely brisk walk. If you don't believe me get on a treadmill and walk at the speed of 4 miles per hour. You're walking at the speed of some of the slowest runners. Just for fun speed up to 5 miles per hour and see how fast the walking is. Don't get injured though!

Finally, finishing for the sake of finishing is the third strategy. This is the easiest strategy because it doesn't matter about time or receiving a medal. If the course closes down, you can still finish your goal. Please remember, if you do decide to go this route that your safety could be in peril if your chip time continues past the course cutoff time.

# Pacing Tables

| Pace Minutes/Mile | Pace Minutes/Km | Half Marathon Finish Times | Marathon Finish Times | Notes |
|---|---|---|---|---|
| 20 (3 mph) | 12:26 | 4:22 | 8:44 | Easy walking pace |
| 19 | 11:49 | 4:09 | 8:18 | Medium walking pace |
| 18 | 11:22 | 3:56 | 7:52 | Medium walking pace |
| 17 | 10:33 | 3:42 | 7:25 | Medium-Fast pace |
| 16 | 9:58 | 3:30 | 7:00 | Fast walking pace |
| 15 (4 mph) | 9:19 | 3:16 | 6:33 | Brisk walking pace |
| 14 | 8:42 | 3:03 | 6:07 | Easy run/walk pace |
| 13 | 8:04 | 2:50 | 5:40 | Medium run/walk pace |
| 12 (5 mph) | 7:27 | 2:37 | 5:14 | Medium run/walk pace |
| 11 | 6:50 | 2:24 | 4:48 | Medium run/walk pace |
| 10 (6 mph) | 6:13 | 2:11 | 4:22 | Runner's pace |

# How long do you have to train for the race?

Determining how long you have to train for a race is an important factor of successfully completing your training schedule. Since you're likely training to walk a half marathon or marathon, you get one advantage over runners that are training for a half marathon or marathon. Depending on your walking assessment you might be able to skip 1, 2, 3 weeks or more. You can't skip during running unless you're already running long distances.

Since your walking your muscles don't require near as much hardening and conditioning as running. Also, your Glycogen stores that keep your energy for your race is depleted at a much slower rate than running. Yes, you are on your feet much longer and your pacing is much slower, however you can easily consume more solid food than runners. Runners must stick to gels and liquids, although some runners do eat whole foods, but not most. Running jostles the food around in your stomach. As walkers, you can eat whatever you like and whatever you can stomach.

You're going to want to invest in a fanny pack or a backpack that you can carry your food during training and on race day. If you don't want to carry food, then you need to have food available on the course. Some people ask their friends or family members to have a pizza or sandwich for them at certain miles of the race.

# Do you have any injuries?

If you're injured and you can't walk for a continuous amount of time such as thirty minutes, then you need to consult a medical professional. I'm not a medical professional nor do I give any type of injury rehabilitation nor assessment of such injuries. There are a few good books and home remedies that could possibly help your injury. However, I haven't tried, nor have I assessed the actual effectiveness of these remedies. Try at your own risk and again your best solution, if you're injured, is to seek a licensed medical professional.

*Running Injury-Free: How to Prevent, Treat, and Recover From Runner's Knee, Shin Splints, Sore Feet and Every Other Ache and Pain* by Joseph Ellis

*Sports Injury Prevention and Rehabilitation* by David Joyce

# Part III - Half Marathons

# Resources on Website

For a free down-loadable PDF of the half marathon and marathon training schedules please visit:

https://halfmarathonforbeginners.com/resources/

# Definitions

The **CT** in the training schedules (located on the following pages) refers to cross training. On **CT days** select an activity other than walking that you enjoy doing. The activity can be anything you want. Most runners/walkers should at least consider weight training one of the days of the week as a cross training exercise. Yoga is another popular choice among runners and walkers. Also, there are two rest days for each week. You don't have to rest both days. If you're feeling OK and don't need to rest, then go ahead and cross train for 30 minutes to 1 hour. I would recommend at the bare minimum that you rest for at least one day a week. Either the day before your long walk or the day after your long walk.

The **REST** in the training schedules is for days you need to rest on. Since you're not running a half marathon or marathon, technically you don't need rest days. If your body feels good, then you can go ahead and cross train on any of the rest days that are on the schedule. If your body is tired and needs to rest then do just that.

# Tips for half marathon training

Remember that your goal for a half marathon race should be to finish within the cutoff time. During your training you need to keep a pace under 20 minutes per mile or 12:26 minutes per kilometer

During your half marathon training you need to practice interval training. On the detailed weekly schedule, I went with Wednesday as the interval training day. Does it have to be on Wednesday? No. You can pick any day to interval train. I highly recommend that your interval train at the bare minimum of 1 day a week. If you feel up to it, then you can interval train on more than one day. Interval training is nothing more than alternating between a fast and slow walking pace. For example, walk 1-minute fast walking followed by 4 minutes casual/regular walking.

Examples of interval training:
- Walk 1-minute fast walking followed by 4 minutes regular walking
- Walk 2 minutes fast walking followed by 3 minutes regular walking
- Walk 2.5 minutes fast walking followed by 2.5 minutes regular walking
- Walk 2 minutes fast walking followed by 8 minutes regular walking.

You are at liberty to design the intervals that you're most comfortable with. Don't forget if you want to run part of the race you can use an interval type system as well.

My training schedules for walking a half marathon spans 12 weeks. Do you have to train the full 12 weeks to walk a half marathon? Absolutely not. Depending on how fit you are, you might be able to forgo several weeks of training. See the previous *Pre-Training Assessment* section to find out where you should start.

# Half Marathon Training Schedules (Miles)

## Walk-A-Thon Half Marathon (miles)

| Week # | Mon. | Tue. | Wed. | Thur. | Fri. | Sat | Sun | Total Miles | Notes |
|---|---|---|---|---|---|---|---|---|---|
| 1 | 4 | CT | 4 | Rest | 4 | 5 | Rest/CT | 17 | |
| 2 | 4 | CT | 4 | Rest | 4 | 6 | Rest/CT | 18 | |
| 3 | 4 | CT | 5 | Rest | 4 | 7 | Rest/CT | 20 | |
| 4 | 4 | CT | 5 | Rest | 4 | 7 | Rest/CT | 20 | |
| 5 | 4 | CT | 5 | Rest | 4 | 8 | Rest/CT | 21 | |
| 6 | 4 | CT | 5 | Rest | 4 | 9 | Rest/CT | 22 | |
| 7 | 4 | CT | 6 | Rest | 4 | 9 | Rest/CT | 23 | |
| 8 | 4 | CT | 7 | Rest | 4 | 10 | Rest/CT | 25 | |
| 9 | 4 | CT | 6 | Rest | 4 | 11 | Rest/CT | 25 | |
| 10 | 4 | CT | 6 | Rest | 4 | 12 | Rest/CT | 26 | |
| 11 | 4 | CT | 6 | Rest | 4 | 8 | Rest/CT | 22 | |
| 12 | 4 | CT | 4 | Rest | 4 | 13.1 Race Day | Rest | 25.1 | |

# Half Marathon Training Schedules (KM)

# Walk-A-Thon Half Marathon (kilometers)

| Week # | Mon. | Tue. | Wed. | Thur. | Fri. | Sat | Sun | Total Miles | Notes |
|--------|------|------|------|-------|------|-----|-----|-------------|-------|
| 1 | 6.4 | CT | 6.4 | Rest | 6.4 | 8 | Rest/CT | 27.2 | |
| 2 | 6.4 | CT | 6.4 | Rest | 6.4 | 9.6 | Rest/CT | 28.8 | |
| 3 | 6.4 | CT | 8 | Rest | 6.4 | 11.2 | Rest/CT | 32 | |
| 4 | 6.4 | CT | 8 | Rest | 6.4 | 11.2 | Rest/CT | 32 | |
| 5 | 6.4 | CT | 8 | Rest | 6.4 | 12.8 | Rest/CT | 33.6 | |
| 6 | 6.4 | CT | 8 | Rest | 6.4 | 14.4 | Rest/CT | 35.2 | |
| 7 | 6.4 | CT | 9.6 | Rest | 6.4 | 14.4 | Rest/CT | 36.8 | |
| 8 | 6.4 | CT | 11.2 | Rest | 6.4 | 16 | Rest/CT | 40 | |
| 9 | 6.4 | CT | 9.6 | Rest | 6.4 | 17.6 | Rest/CT | 40 | |
| 10 | 6.4 | CT | 9.6 | Rest | 6.4 | 19.2 | Rest/CT | 41.6 | |
| 11 | 6.4 | CT | 9.6 | Rest | 6.4 | 12.8 | Rest/CT | 35.2 | |
| 12 | 6.4 | CT | 6.4 | Rest | 6.4 | 21 Race Day | Rest | 40.2 | |

# Half Marathon Training - Week 1

| Mon | 4 miles (6.4 km) | Rest. Take it easy. Don't walk. If you need to exercise, I recommend a walk for no longer than 30 minutes. |
|---|---|---|
| Tue | CT 30 minutes | Cross train in an activity that complements your walking. Try not to walk since you're already walking during you're normal training schedule. Try biking, yoga, weights, spin class, pump-it-up group class, etc. |
| Wed | 4 miles (6.4 km) | Perfect day to practice interval training. For example, walk at your goal race pace for 4 minutes and then speed up your pace for 1 minute. Repeat until you complete the distance for the day. You can change your intervals as well such as 3 minutes walking at goal race pace and 2 minutes walking briskly. Or you could walk 9 minutes goal race pace and walk 1 minute briskly. |
| Thu | Rest | Do as little activity as possible. Fridays are important rest days. In order for your muscles to grow stronger they need rest. |
| Fri | 4 miles (6.4 km) | Walk at your goal race pace. |

| Sat | 5 miles (8 km) | The most important part of your long duration walks is finishing the distance. Attempt to walk these at your half marathon goal race pace. This week the distance is not too far. As the weeks continue, the distance required to walk becomes greater and greater. As the long duration walks continue to gradually increase, you might not be able to keep goal race pace. If this happens, don't sweat it, do the best you can and finish the distance. You're far better off to finish the distance at a slower pace than quit walking altogether because you're tired. |
| Sun | Rest/CT 30 minutes | Rest or cross train. Since you're not planning on running the half marathon, you could easily cross train for thirty minutes in the activity of your choice. |
| **Notes** | | |
| | | |

- Get plenty of sleep the night before your long duration walk.
- Try to walk your long duration walk early in the morning.
- After each walk it's important to stretch out your muscles.

# Half Marathon Training - Week 2

| Mon | 4 miles (6.4 km) | Rest. Take it easy. Don't walk. If you need to exercise, I recommend a walk for no longer than 30 minutes. |
|---|---|---|
| Tue | CT 30 minutes | Cross train in an activity that complements your walking. Try not to walk since you're already walking during your normal training schedule. Try biking, yoga, weights, spin class, pump-it-up group class, etc. |
| Wed | 4 miles (6.4 km) | Perfect day to practice interval training. For example, walk at your goal race pace for 4 minutes and then speed up your pace for 1 minute. Repeat until you complete the distance for the day. You can change your intervals as well such as 3 minutes walking at goal race pace and 2 minutes walking briskly. Or you could walk 9 minutes goal race pace and walk 1 minute briskly. |
| Thu | Rest | Do as little activity as possible. Fridays are important rest days. In order for your muscles to grow stronger they need rest. |
| Fri | 4 miles (6.4 km) | Walk at your goal race pace. |

| Sat | 6 miles (9.6 km) | The most important part of your long duration walks is finishing the distance. Attempt to walk these at your half marathon goal race pace. This week the distance is not too far. As the weeks continue, the distance required to walk becomes greater and greater. As the long duration walks continue to gradually increase, you might not be able to keep goal race pace. If this happens, don't sweat it, do the best you can and finish the distance. You're far better off to finish the distance at a slower pace than quit walking altogether because you're tired. |
|-----|------------------|------------------------------------------------------------------------------------------------------------------------------------------------------------------------------------------------------------------------------------------------------------------------------------------------------------------------------------------------------------------------------------------------------------------------------------------------------------------------------------------------------------------------------------------------|
| Sun | Rest/CT 30 minutes | Rest or cross train. Since you're not planning on running the half marathon, you could easily cross train for thirty minutes in the activity of your choice. |
| **Notes** | | |
| | | |

- Get plenty of sleep the night before your long duration walk.
- Try to walk your long duration walk early in the morning.
- After each walk it's important to stretch out your muscles.

# Half Marathon Training - Week 3

| Mon | 4 miles (6.4 km) | Rest. Take it easy. Don't walk. If you need to exercise, I recommend a walk for no longer than 30 minutes. |
|---|---|---|
| Tue | CT 30 minutes | Cross train in an activity that complements your walking. Try not to walk since you're already walking during your normal training schedule. Try biking, yoga, weights, spin class, pump-it-up group class, etc. |
| Wed | 5 miles (8 km) | Perfect day to practice interval training. For example, walk at your goal race pace for 4 minutes and then speed up your pace for 1 minute. Repeat until you complete the distance for the day. You can change your intervals as well such as 3 minutes walking at goal race pace and 2 minutes walking briskly. Or you could walk 9 minutes goal race pace and walk 1 minute briskly. |
| Thu | Rest | Do as little activity as possible. Fridays are important rest days. In order for your muscles to grow stronger they need rest. |
| Fri | 4 miles (6.4 km) | Walk at your goal race pace. |

| Sat | 7 miles (11.2 km) | The most important part of your long duration walks is finishing the distance. Attempt to walk these at your half marathon goal race pace. This week the distance is not too far. As the weeks continue, the distance required to walk becomes greater and greater. As the long duration walks continue to gradually increase, you might not be able to keep goal race pace. If this happens, don't sweat it, do the best you can and finish the distance. You're far better off to finish the distance at a slower pace than quit walking altogether because you're tired. |
|-----|-------------------|---|
| Sun | Rest/CT 30 minutes | Rest or cross train. Since you're not planning on running the half marathon, you could easily cross train for thirty minutes in the activity of your choice. |
| **Notes** | | |
| | | |

- Get plenty of sleep the night before your long duration walk.
- Try to walk your long duration walk early in the morning.
- After each walk it's important to stretch out your muscles.

# Half Marathon Training - Week 4

| Mon | 4 miles (6.4 km) | Rest. Take it easy. Don't walk. If you need to exercise, I recommend a walk for no longer than 30 minutes. |
|---|---|---|
| Tue | CT 30 minutes | Cross train in an activity that complements your walking. Try not to walk since you're already walking during your normal training schedule. Try biking, yoga, weights, spin class, pump-it-up group class, etc. |
| Wed | 5 miles (8 km) | Perfect day to practice interval training. For example, walk at your goal race pace for 4 minutes and then speed up your pace for 1 minute. Repeat until you complete the distance for the day. You can change your intervals as well such as 3 minutes walking at goal race pace and 2 minutes walking briskly. Or you could walk 9 minutes goal race pace and walk 1 minute briskly. |
| Thu | Rest | Do as little activity as possible. Fridays are important rest days. In order for your muscles to grow stronger they need rest. |
| Fri | 4 miles (6.4 km) | Walk at your goal race pace. |

| Sat | 7 miles (11.2 km) | The most important part of your long duration walks is finishing the distance. Attempt to walk these at your half marathon goal race pace. This week the distance is not too far. As the weeks continue, the distance required to walk becomes greater and greater. As the long duration walks continue to gradually increase, you might not be able to keep goal race pace. If this happens, don't sweat it, do the best you can and finish the distance. You're far better off to finish the distance at a slower pace than quit walking altogether because you're tired. |
|---|---|---|
| Sun | Rest/CT 30 minutes | Rest or cross train. Since you're not planning on running the half marathon, you could easily cross train for thirty minutes in the activity of your choice. |

### Notes

<br><br><br><br>

- Get plenty of sleep the night before your long duration walk.
- Try to walk your long duration walk early in the morning.
- After each walk it's important to stretch out your muscles.

# Half Marathon Training - Week 5

| Mon | 4 miles (6.4 km) | Rest. Take it easy. Don't walk. If you need to exercise, I recommend a walk for no longer than 30 minutes. |
|---|---|---|
| Tue | CT 30 minutes | Cross train in an activity that complements your walking. Try not to walk since you're already walking during your normal training schedule. Try biking, yoga, weights, spin class, pump-it-up group class, etc. |
| Wed | 5 miles (8 km) | Perfect day to practice interval training. For example, walk at your goal race pace for 4 minutes and then speed up your pace for 1 minute. Repeat until you complete the distance for the day. You can change your intervals as well such as 3 minutes walking at goal race pace and 2 minutes walking briskly. Or you could walk 9 minutes goal race pace and walk 1 minute briskly. |
| Thu | Rest | Do as little activity as possible. Fridays are important rest days. In order for your muscles to grow stronger they need rest. |
| Fri | 4 miles (6.4 km) | Walk at your goal race pace. |

| Sat | 8 miles (12.8 km) | The most important part of your long duration walks is finishing the distance. Attempt to walk these at your half marathon goal race pace. This week the distance is not too far. As the weeks continue, the distance required to walk becomes greater and greater. As the long duration walks continue to gradually increase, you might not be able to keep goal race pace. If this happens, don't sweat it, do the best you can and finish the distance. You're far better off to finish the distance at a slower pace than quit walking altogether because you're tired. |
|-----|-----|-----|
| Sun | Rest/CT 30 minutes | Rest or cross train. Since you're not planning on running the half marathon, you could easily cross train for thirty minutes in the activity of your choice. |
| **Notes** | | |
|  | | |

- Get plenty of sleep the night before your long duration walk.
- Try to walk your long duration walk early in the morning.
- After each walk it's important to stretch out your muscles.

# Half Marathon Training - Week 6

| Mon | 4 miles (6.4 km) | Rest. Take it easy. Don't walk. If you need to exercise, I recommend a walk for no longer than 30 minutes. |
|---|---|---|
| Tue | CT 30 minutes | Cross train in an activity that complements your walking. Try not to walk since you're already walking during your normal training schedule. Try biking, yoga, weights, spin class, pump-it-up group class, etc. |
| Wed | 5 miles (8 km) | Perfect day to practice interval training. For example, walk at your goal race pace for 4 minutes and then speed up your pace for 1 minute. Repeat until you complete the distance for the day. You can change your intervals as well such as 3 minutes walking at goal race pace and 2 minutes walking briskly. Or you could walk 9 minutes goal race pace and walk 1 minute briskly. |
| Thu | Rest | Do as little activity as possible. Fridays are important rest days. In order for your muscles to grow stronger they need rest. |
| Fri | 4 miles (6.4 km) | Walk at your goal race pace. |

| Sat | 9 miles (14.4 km) | The most important part of your long duration walks is finishing the distance. Attempt to walk these at your half marathon goal race pace. This week's distance is closing in on a walk that might last over 3 hours. As the weeks continue, the distance required to walk becomes greater and greater. As the long duration walks continue to gradually increase, you might not be able to keep goal race pace. If this happens, don't sweat it, do the best you can and finish the distance. You're far better off to finish the distance at a slower pace than quit walking altogether because you're tired. |
|-----|-------|---------------------------------------------|
| Sun | Rest/CT 30 minutes | Rest or cross train. Since you're not planning on running the half marathon, you could easily cross train for thirty minutes in the activity of your choice. |
| **Notes** || |
|  || |

- Get plenty of sleep the night before your long duration walk.
- Try to walk your long duration walk early in the morning.
- After each walk it's important to stretch out your muscles.
- If your long walks are taking up too much time, consider splitting up your walks into two different sessions possibly one in the morning and one at night.

# Half Marathon Training - Week 7

| Mon | 4 miles (6.4 km) | Rest. Take it easy. Don't walk. If you need to exercise, I recommend a walk for no longer than 30 minutes. |
|---|---|---|
| Tue | CT 30 minutes | Cross train in an activity that complements your walking. Try not to walk since you're already walking during your normal training schedule. Try biking, yoga, weights, spin class, pump-it-up group class, etc. |
| Wed | 6 miles (9.6 km) | Perfect day to practice interval training. For example, walk at your goal race pace for 4 minutes and then speed up your pace for 1 minute. Repeat until you complete the distance for the day. You can change your intervals as well such as 3 minutes walking at goal race pace and 2 minutes walking briskly. Or you could walk 9 minutes goal race pace and walk 1 minute briskly. |
| Thu | Rest | Do as little activity as possible. Fridays are important rest days. In order for your muscles to grow stronger they need rest. |
| Fri | 4 miles (6.4 km) | Walk at your goal race pace. |

| Sat | 9 miles (14.4 km) | The most important part of your long duration walks is finishing the distance. Attempt to walk these at your half marathon goal race pace. This week's distance is closing in on a walk that might last over 3 hours. As the weeks continue, the distance required to walk becomes greater and greater. As the long duration walks continue to gradually increase, you might not be able to keep goal race pace. If this happens, don't sweat it, do the best you can and finish the distance. You're far better off to finish the distance at a slower pace than quit walking altogether because you're tired. |
|---|---|---|
| Sun | Rest/CT 30 minutes | Rest or cross train. Since you're not planning on running the half marathon, you could easily cross train for thirty minutes in the activity of your choice. |
| **Notes** | | |
| | | |

- Get plenty of sleep the night before your long duration walk.
- Try to walk your long duration walk early in the morning.
- After each walk it's important to stretch out your muscles.
- If your long walks are taking up too much time, consider splitting up your long-distance walks into two different sessions possibly one in the morning and one at night.

# Half Marathon Training - Week 8

| | | |
|---|---|---|
| Mon | 4 miles (6.4 km) | Rest. Take it easy. Don't walk. If you need to exercise, I recommend a walk for no longer than 30 minutes. |
| Tue | CT 30 minutes | Cross train in an activity that complements your walking. Try not to walk since you're already walking during your normal training schedule. Try biking, yoga, weights, spin class, pump-it-up group class, etc. |
| Wed | 7 miles (11.2 km) | Perfect day to practice interval training. For example, walk at your goal race pace for 4 minutes and then speed up your pace for 1 minute. Repeat until you complete the distance for the day. You can change your intervals as well such as 3 minutes walking at goal race pace and 2 minutes walking briskly. Or you could walk 9 minutes goal race pace and walk 1 minute briskly. |
| Thu | Rest | Do as little activity as possible. Fridays are important rest days. In order for your muscles to grow stronger they need rest. |
| Fri | 4 miles (6.4 km) | Walk at your goal race pace. |

| Sat | 10 miles (16 km) | The most important part of your long duration walks is finishing the distance. Attempt to walk these at your half marathon goal race pace. This week's distance is closing in on a walk that might last over 3 hours. As the weeks continue, the distance required to walk becomes greater and greater. As the long duration walks continue to gradually increase, you might not be able to keep goal race pace. If this happens, don't sweat it, do the best you can and finish the distance. You're far better off to finish the distance at a slower pace than quit walking altogether because you're tired. |
|-----|------------------|-----------------------------------------------------------------------------------------------------------------------------------------------------------------------------------------------------------------------------------------------------------------------------------------------------------------------------------------------------------------------------------------------------------------------------------------------------------------------------------------------------------------------------------------------------------------------------------------------------------------------------------------------------------------------------------------------------------------------------------|
| Sun | Rest/CT 30 minutes | Rest or cross train. Since you're not planning on running the half marathon, you could easily cross train for thirty minutes in the activity of your choice. |
| **Notes** | | |
|  | | |

- Get plenty of sleep the night before your long duration walk.
- Try to walk your long duration walk early in the morning.
- After each walk it's important to stretch out your muscles.
- If your long walks are taking up too much time, consider splitting up your walks into two different sessions possibly one in the morning and one at night.

# Half Marathon Training - Week 9

| Mon | 4 miles (6.4 km) | Rest. Take it easy. Don't walk. If you need to exercise, I recommend a walk for no longer than 30 minutes. |
|---|---|---|
| Tue | CT 30 minutes | Cross train in an activity that complements your walking. Try not to walk since you're already walking during your normal training schedule. Try biking, yoga, weights, spin class, pump-it-up group class, etc. |
| Wed | 6 miles (9.6 km) | Perfect day to practice interval training. For example, walk at your goal race pace for 4 minutes and then speed up your pace for 1 minute. Repeat until you complete the distance for the day. You can change your intervals as well such as 3 minutes walking at goal race pace and 2 minutes walking briskly. Or you could walk 9 minutes goal race pace and walk 1 minute briskly. |
| Thu | Rest | Do as little activity as possible. Fridays are important rest days. In order for your muscles to grow stronger they need rest. |
| Fri | 4 miles (6.4 km) | Walk at your goal race pace. |

| Sat | 11 miles (17.6 km) | The most important part of your long duration walks is finishing the distance. Attempt to walk these at your half marathon goal race pace. This week's distance is closing in on a walk that might last over 3 hours. As the weeks continue, the distance required to walk becomes greater and greater. As the long duration walks continue to gradually increase, you might not be able to keep goal race pace. If this happens, don't sweat it, do the best you can and finish the distance. You're far better off to finish the distance at a slower pace than quit walking altogether because you're tired. |
|-----|--------------------|---|
| Sun | Rest/CT 30 minutes | Rest or cross train. Since you're not planning on running the half marathon, you could easily cross train for thirty minutes in the activity of your choice. |
| **Notes** | | |
| | | |

- Get plenty of sleep the night before your long duration walk.
- Try to walk your long duration walk early in the morning.
- After each walk it's important to stretch out your muscles.
- If your long walks are taking up too much time, consider splitting up your walks into two different sessions possibly one in the morning and one at night.

# Half Marathon Training - Week 10

| Mon | 4 miles (6.4 km) | Rest. Take it easy. Don't walk. If you need to exercise, I recommend a walk for no longer than 30 minutes. |
|---|---|---|
| Tue | CT 30 minutes | Cross train in an activity that complements your walking. Try not to walk since you're already walking during your normal training schedule. Try biking, yoga, weights, spin class, pump-it-up group class, etc. |
| Wed | 6 miles (9.6 km) | Perfect day to practice interval training. For example, walk at your goal race pace for 4 minutes and then speed up your pace for 1 minute. Repeat until you complete the distance for the day. You can change your intervals as well such as 3 minutes walking at goal race pace and 2 minutes walking briskly. Or you could walk 9 minutes goal race pace and walk 1 minute briskly. |
| Thu | Rest | Do as little activity as possible. Fridays are important rest days. In order for your muscles to grow stronger they need rest. |
| Fri | 4 miles (6.4 km) | Walk at your goal race pace. |

| Sat | 12 miles (19.2 km) | The most important part of your long duration walks is finishing the distance. Attempt to walk these at your half marathon goal race pace. This week's distance is closing in on a walk that might last over 3 hours. As the weeks continue, the distance required to walk becomes greater and greater. As the long duration walks continue to gradually increase, you might not be able to keep goal race pace. If this happens, don't sweat it, do the best you can and finish the distance. You're far better off to finish the distance at a slower pace than quit walking altogether because you're tired. |
|-----|------|------|
| Sun | Rest/CT 30 minutes | Rest or cross train. Since you're not planning on running the half marathon, you could easily cross train for thirty minutes in the activity of your choice. |
| **Notes** | | |
| | | |

- Get plenty of sleep the night before your long duration walk.
- Try to walk your long duration walk early in the morning.
- After each walk it's important to stretch out your muscles.
- If your long walks are taking up too much time, consider splitting up your walks into two different sessions possibly one in the morning and one at night.

# Half Marathon Training - Week 11

| | | |
|---|---|---|
| Mon | 4 miles (6.4 km) | Rest. Take it easy. Don't walk. If you need to exercise, I recommend a walk for no longer than 30 minutes. |
| Tue | CT 30 minutes | Cross train in an activity that complements your walking. Try not to walk since you're already walking during your normal training schedule. Try biking, yoga, weights, spin class, pump-it-up group class, etc. |
| Wed | 6 miles (9.6 km) | Perfect day to practice interval training. For example, walk at your goal race pace for 4 minutes and then speed up your pace for 1 minute. Repeat until you complete the distance for the day. You can change your intervals as well such as 3 minutes walking at goal race pace and 2 minutes walking briskly. Or you could walk 9 minutes goal race pace and walk 1 minute briskly. |
| Thu | Rest | Do as little activity as possible. Fridays are important rest days. In order for your muscles to grow stronger they need rest. |
| Fri | 4 miles (6.4 km) | Walk at your goal race pace. |

| Sat | 8 miles (12.8 km) | The most important part of your long duration walks is finishing the distance. Attempt to walk these at your half marathon goal race pace. This week's distance is closing in on a walk that might last over 3 hours. As the weeks continue, the distance required to walk becomes greater and greater. As the long duration walks continue to gradually increase, you might not be able to keep goal race pace. If this happens, don't sweat it, do the best you can and finish the distance. You're far better off to finish the distance at a slower pace than quit walking altogether because you're tired. |
| Sun | Rest/CT 30 minutes | Rest or cross train. Since you're not planning on running the half marathon, you could easily cross train for thirty minutes in the activity of your choice. |
| **Notes** | | |
| | | |

- Get plenty of sleep the night before your long duration walk.
- Try to walk your long duration walk early in the morning.
- After each walk it's important to stretch out your muscles.
- If your long walks are taking up too much time, consider splitting up your walks into two different sessions possibly one in the morning and one at night.

# Half Marathon Training - Week 12

| | | |
|---|---|---|
| Mon | 4 miles (6.4 km) | Walk at your goal race pace. |
| Tue | CT 30 minutes | Cross train in an activity that complements your walking. Try not to walk since you're already walking during your normal training schedule. Try biking, yoga, weights, spin class, pump-it-up group class, etc. |
| Wed | 4 miles (6.4 km) | Walk at your goal race pace. |
| Thu | Rest | Do as little activity as possible. Fridays are important rest days. In order for your muscles to grow stronger they need rest. |
| Fri | 4 miles (6.4 km) | Walk at your goal race pace. |
| Sat | 13.1 miles (21 km) | RACE DAY! |
| Sun | Rest | Rest and celebrate your victory! |

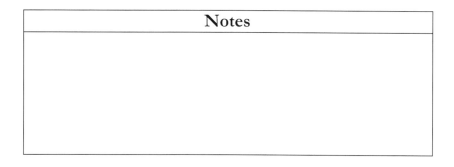

- Get plenty of sleep the night before your long duration walk.
- Try to walk your long duration walk early in the morning.
- After each walk it's important to stretch out your muscles.
- If your long walks are taking up too much time, consider splitting up your walks into two different sessions possibly one in the morning and one at night.
- This week your body needs as much rest as possible.

# Part IV – Marathon

# Definitions

The **CT** in the training schedules (located on the following pages) refers to cross training. On **CT days** select an activity other than walking that you enjoy doing. The activity can be anything you want. Most runners/walkers should at least consider weight training one of the days of the week as a cross training exercise. Yoga is another popular choice among runners and walkers. Also, there are two rest days for each week. You don't have to rest both days. If you're feeling OK and don't need to rest, then go ahead and cross train for 30 minutes to 1 hour. I would recommend at the bare minimum that you rest for at least one day a week. Either the day before your long walk or the day after your long walk.

The **REST** in the training schedules is for days you need to rest on. Since you're not running a half marathon or marathon, technically you don't need rest days. If your body feels good, then you can go ahead and cross train on any of the rest days that are on the schedule. If your body is tired and needs to rest, then do just that.

The **HM Race 13.1** on the marathon training schedule is optional. If you want to get an extra race in, then go for it. If you just want to log miles walking, then do that instead. Also, the timing of the HM Race 13.1 on the schedule can be moved around as necessary, it's not written in stone that you must perform this on week 10.

# Tips for marathon training

Remember that your goal for a marathon race should be to finish within the cutoff time.

During your training you need to keep a pace under 20 minutes per mile or 12:26 minutes per kilometer

During your marathon training you need to practice interval training. On the detailed weekly schedule, I went with Wednesday as the interval training day. Does it have to be on Wednesday? No. You can pick any day to interval train. I highly recommend that your interval train at the bare minimum of at least 1 day per week. If you feel up to it, then you can interval train on more than one day. Interval training is nothing more than alternating between a fast and slow walking pace. For example, walk 1-minute fast walking followed by 4 minutes casual/regular walking.

Examples of interval training:
- Walk 1-minute fast walking followed by 4 minutes regular walking
- Walk 2 minutes fast walking followed by 3 minutes regular walking
- Walk 2.5 minutes fast walking followed by 2.5 minutes regular walking
- Walk 2 minutes fast walking followed by 8 minutes regular walking.

You are at liberty to design the intervals that you're most comfortable with. Don't forget if you want to run part of the race you can use an interval type system as well.

My training schedules for walking a marathon spans 18 weeks. Do you have to train the full 18 weeks to walk a half marathon? Absolutely not. Depending on how fit you are, you might be able to forgo several weeks of training. See the previous *Pre-Training Assessment* section to find out where you should start.

# Marathon Training Schedules (Miles)

## Walk-A-Thon Marathon (miles)

| Week # | Mon. | Tue. | Wed. | Thur. | Fri. | Sat | Sun | Total Miles | Notes |
|--------|------|------|------|-------|------|-----|-----|-------------|-------|
| 1 | 4 | CT | 4 | Rest | 4 | 6 | Rest/CT | 18 | |
| 2 | 4 | CT | 4 | Rest | 4 | 7 | Rest/CT | 19 | |
| 3 | 4 | CT | 4 | Rest | 4 | 8 | Rest/CT | 20 | |
| 4 | 4 | CT | 6 | Rest | 4 | 9 | Rest/CT | 23 | |
| 5 | 4 | CT | 6 | Rest | 4 | 10 | Rest/CT | 24 | |
| 6 | 4 | CT | 6 | Rest | 4 | 11 | Rest/CT | 25 | |
| 7 | 4 | CT | 8 | Rest | 4 | 12 | Rest/CT | 28 | |
| 8 | 6 | CT | 8 | Rest | 4 | 14 | Rest/CT | 32 | |
| 9 | 6 | CT | 8 | Rest | 4 | 16 | Rest/CT | 34 | |
| 10 | 4 | CT | 4 | Rest | 4 | HM Race 13.1 | Rest/CT | 25.1 | |
| 11 | 6 | CT | 6 | Rest | 4 | 14 | Rest/CT | 30 | |
| 12 | 6 | CT | 8 | Rest | 4 | 16 | Rest/CT | 34 | |
| 13 | 8 | CT | 10 | Rest | 4 | 18 | Rest/CT | 40 | |
| 14 | 6 | CT | 10 | Rest | 4 | 20 | Rest/CT | 40 | |
| 15 | 8 | CT | 10 | Rest | 4 | 22 | Rest/CT | 44 | |
| 16 | 6 | CT | 8 | Rest | 4 | 18 | Rest/CT | 36 | |
| 17 | 4 | CT | 6 | Rest | 4 | 12 | Rest/CT | 26 | |
| 18 | 6.4 | 6 | 4 | Rest | Rest | RACE 26.2 | Rest | 40.2 | |

# Marathon Training Schedules (KM)

## Walk-A-Thon Marathon (kilometers)

| Week # | Mon. | Tue. | Wed. | Thur. | Fri. | Sat | Sun | Total Miles | Notes |
|--------|------|------|------|-------|------|-----|-----|-------------|-------|
| 1 | 6.4 | CT | 6.4 | Rest | 6.4 | 9.6 | Rest/CT | 28.8 | |
| 2 | 6.4 | CT | 6.4 | Rest | 6.4 | 11.2 | Rest/CT | 30.4 | |
| 3 | 6.4 | CT | 6.4 | Rest | 6.4 | 12.8 | Rest/CT | 32 | |
| 4 | 6.4 | CT | 9.6 | Rest | 6.4 | 14.4 | Rest/CT | 36.8 | |
| 5 | 6.4 | CT | 9.6 | Rest | 6.4 | 16 | Rest/CT | 38.4 | |
| 6 | 6.4 | CT | 9.6 | Rest | 6.4 | 17.6 | Rest/CT | 40 | |
| 7 | 6.4 | CT | 12.8 | Rest | 6.4 | 19.2 | Rest/CT | 44.8 | |
| 8 | 9.6 | CT | 12.8 | Rest | 6.4 | 22.4 | Rest/CT | 51.2 | |
| 9 | 9.6 | CT | 12.8 | Rest | 6.4 | 25.6 | Rest/CT | 54.4 | |
| 10 | 6.4 | CT | 6.4 | Rest | 6.4 | HM Race 21 | Rest/CT | 40.2 | |
| 11 | 9.6 | CT | 9.6 | Rest | 6.4 | 22.4 | Rest/CT | 48 | |
| 12 | 9.6 | CT | 12.8 | Rest | 6.4 | 25.6 | Rest/CT | 54.4 | |
| 13 | 12.8 | CT | 16 | Rest | 6.4 | 28.8 | Rest/CT | 64 | |
| 14 | 9.6 | CT | 16 | Rest | 6.4 | 32 | Rest/CT | 64 | |
| 15 | 12.8 | CT | 16 | Rest | 6.4 | 35.2 | Rest/CT | 70.4 | |
| 16 | 9.6 | CT | 12.8 | Rest | 6.4 | 28.8 | Rest/CT | 57.6 | |
| 17 | 6.4 | CT | 9.6 | Rest | 6.4 | 19.2 | Rest/CT | 42 | |
| 18 | 6.4 | 9.6 | 6.4 | Rest | Rest | RACE 42 | Rest | 64.4 | |

# Marathon Training - Week 1

| | | |
|---|---|---|
| Mon | 4 miles (6.4 km) | Rest. Take it easy. Don't walk. If you need to exercise, I recommend a walk for no longer than 30 minutes. |
| Tue | CT 30 minutes | Cross train in an activity that complements your walking. Try not to walk since you're already walking during your normal training schedule. Try biking, yoga, weights, spin class, pump-it-up group class, etc. |
| Wed | 4 miles (6.4 km) | Perfect day to practice interval training. For example, walk at your goal race pace for 4 minutes and then speed up your pace for 1 minute. Repeat until you complete the distance for the day. You can change your intervals as well such as 3 minutes walking at goal race pace and 2 minutes walking briskly. Or you could walk 9 minutes goal race pace and walk 1 minute briskly. |
| Thu | Rest | Do as little activity as possible. Fridays are important rest days. In order for your muscles to grow stronger they need rest. |
| Fri | 4 miles (6.4 km) | Walk at your goal race pace. |

| Sat | 6 miles (9.6 km) | The most important part of your long duration walks is finishing the distance. Attempt to walk these at your half marathon goal race pace. This week the distance is not too far. As the weeks continue, the distance required to walk becomes greater and greater. As the long duration walks continue to gradually increase, you might not be able to keep goal race pace. If this happens, don't sweat it, do the best you can and finish the distance. You're far better off to finish the distance at a slower pace than quit walking altogether because you're tired. |
| Sun | Rest/CT 30 minutes | Rest or cross train. Since you're not planning on running the half marathon, you could easily cross train for thirty minutes in the activity of your choice. |
| **Notes** | | |
|  | | |

- Get plenty of sleep the night before your long duration walk.
- Try to walk your long duration walk early in the morning.
- After each walk it's important to stretch out your muscles.

# Marathon Training - Week 2

| Mon | 4 miles (6.4 km) | Rest. Take it easy. Don't walk. If you need to exercise, I recommend a walk for no longer than 30 minutes. |
|---|---|---|
| Tue | CT 30 minutes | Cross train in an activity that complements your walking. Try not to walk since you're already walking during your normal training schedule. Try biking, yoga, weights, spin class, pump-it-up group class, etc. |
| Wed | 4 miles (6.4 km) | Perfect day to practice interval training. For example, walk at your goal race pace for 4 minutes and then speed up your pace for 1 minute. Repeat until you complete the distance for the day. You can change your intervals as well such as 3 minutes walking at goal race pace and 2 minutes walking briskly. Or you could walk 9 minutes goal race pace and walk 1 minute briskly. |
| Thu | Rest | Do as little activity as possible. Fridays are important rest days. In order for your muscles to grow stronger they need rest. |
| Fri | 4 miles (6.4 km) | Walk at your goal race pace. |

| Sat | 7 miles (11.2 km) | The most important part of your long duration walks is finishing the distance. Attempt to walk these at your half marathon goal race pace. This week the distance is not too far. As the weeks continue, the distance required to walk becomes greater and greater. As the long duration walks continue to gradually increase, you might not be able to keep goal race pace. If this happens, don't sweat it, do the best you can and finish the distance. You're far better off to finish the distance at a slower pace than quit walking altogether because you're tired. |
|-----|-------------------|---|
| Sun | Rest/CT 30 minutes | Rest or cross train. Since you're not planning on running the half marathon, you could easily cross train for thirty minutes in the activity of your choice. |
| **Notes** | | |
| | | |

- Get plenty of sleep the night before your long duration walk.
- Try to walk your long duration walk early in the morning.
- After each walk it's important to stretch out your muscles.

# Marathon Training - Week 3

| Mon | 4 miles (6.4 km) | Rest. Take it easy. Don't walk. If you need to exercise, I recommend a walk for no longer than 30 minutes. |
|---|---|---|
| Tue | CT 30 minutes | Cross train in an activity that complements your walking. Try not to walk since you're already walking during your normal training schedule. Try biking, yoga, weights, spin class, pump-it-up group class, etc. |
| Wed | 4 miles (6.4 km) | Perfect day to practice interval training. For example, walk at your goal race pace for 4 minutes and then speed up your pace for 1 minute. Repeat until you complete the distance for the day. You can change your intervals as well such as 3 minutes walking at goal race pace and 2 minutes walking briskly. Or you could walk 9 minutes goal race pace and walk 1 minute briskly. |
| Thu | Rest | Do as little activity as possible. Fridays are important rest days. In order for your muscles to grow stronger they need rest. |
| Fri | 4 miles (6.4 km) | Walk at your goal race pace. |

| | | |
|---|---|---|
| Sat | 8 miles (12.8 km) | The most important part of your long duration walks is finishing the distance. Attempt to walk these at your half marathon goal race pace. This week the distance is not too far. As the weeks continue, the distance required to walk becomes greater and greater. As the long duration walks continue to gradually increase, you might not be able to keep goal race pace. If this happens, don't sweat it, do the best you can and finish the distance. You're far better off to finish the distance at a slower pace than quit walking altogether because you're tired. |
| Sun | Rest/CT 30 minutes | Rest or cross train. Since you're not planning on running the half marathon, you could easily cross train for thirty minutes in the activity of your choice. |
| **Notes** | | |
| | | |

- Get plenty of sleep the night before your long duration walk.
- Try to walk your long duration walk early in the morning.
- After each walk it's important to stretch out your muscles.

# Marathon Training - Week 4

| Mon | 4 miles (6.4 km) | Rest. Take it easy. Don't walk. If you need to exercise, I recommend a walk for no longer than 30 minutes. |
|---|---|---|
| Tue | CT 30 minutes | Cross train in an activity that complements your walking. Try not to walk since you're already walking during your normal training schedule. Try biking, yoga, weights, spin class, pump-it-up group class, etc. |
| Wed | 6 miles (9.6 km) | Perfect day to practice interval training. For example, walk at your goal race pace for 4 minutes and then speed up your pace for 1 minute. Repeat until you complete the distance for the day. You can change your intervals as well such as 3 minutes walking at goal race pace and 2 minutes walking briskly. Or you could walk 9 minutes goal race pace and walk 1 minute briskly. |
| Thu | Rest | Do as little activity as possible. Fridays are important rest days. In order for your muscles to grow stronger they need rest. |
| Fri | 4 miles (6.4 km) | Walk at your goal race pace. |

| Sat | 9 miles (14.4 km) | The most important part of your long duration walks is finishing the distance. Attempt to walk these at your half marathon goal race pace. This week the distance is not too far. As the weeks continue, the distance required to walk becomes greater and greater. As the long duration walks continue to gradually increase, you might not be able to keep goal race pace. If this happens, don't sweat it, do the best you can and finish the distance. You're far better off to finish the distance at a slower pace than quit walking altogether because you're tired. |
| Sun | Rest/CT 30 minutes | Rest or cross train. Since you're not planning on running the half marathon, you could easily cross train for thirty minutes in the activity of your choice. |
| **Notes** | | |
| | | |

- Get plenty of sleep the night before your long duration walk.
- Try to walk your long duration walk early in the morning.
- After each walk it's important to stretch out your muscles.

# Marathon Training - Week 5

| Mon | 4 miles (6.4 km) | Rest. Take it easy. Don't walk. If you need to exercise, I recommend a walk for no longer than 30 minutes. |
|---|---|---|
| Tue | CT 30 minutes | Cross train in an activity that complements your walking. Try not to walk since you're already walking during your normal training schedule. Try biking, yoga, weights, spin class, pump-it-up group class, etc. |
| Wed | 6 miles (9.6 km) | Perfect day to practice interval training. For example, walk at your goal race pace for 4 minutes and then speed up your pace for 1 minute. Repeat until you complete the distance for the day. You can change your intervals as well such as 3 minutes walking at goal race pace and 2 minutes walking briskly. Or you could walk 9 minutes goal race pace and walk 1 minute briskly. |
| Thu | Rest | Do as little activity as possible. Fridays are important rest days. In order for your muscles to grow stronger they need rest. |
| Fri | 4 miles (6.4 km) | Walk at your goal race pace. |

| Sat | 10 miles (16 km) | The most important part of your long duration walks is finishing the distance. Attempt to walk these at your half marathon goal race pace. This week the distance is not too far. As the weeks continue, the distance required to walk becomes greater and greater. As the long duration walks continue to gradually increase, you might not be able to keep goal race pace. If this happens, don't sweat it, do the best you can and finish the distance. You're far better off to finish the distance at a slower pace than quit walking altogether because you're tired. |
| Sun | Rest/CT 30 minutes | Rest or cross train. Since you're not planning on running the half marathon, you could easily cross train for thirty minutes in the activity of your choice. |
| **Notes** | | |
| | | |

- Get plenty of sleep the night before your long duration walk.
- Try to walk your long duration walk early in the morning.
- After each walk it's important to stretch out your muscles.

# Marathon Training - Week 6

| Mon | 4 miles (6.4 km) | Rest. Take it easy. Don't walk. If you need to exercise, I recommend a walk for no longer than 30 minutes. |
|---|---|---|
| Tue | CT 30 minutes | Cross train in an activity that complements your walking. Try not to walk since you're already walking during your normal training schedule. Try biking, yoga, weights, spin class, pump-it-up group class, etc. |
| Wed | 6 miles (9.6 km) | Perfect day to practice interval training. For example, walk at your goal race pace for 4 minutes and then speed up your pace for 1 minute. Repeat until you complete the distance for the day. You can change your intervals as well such as 3 minutes walking at goal race pace and 2 minutes walking briskly. Or you could walk 9 minutes goal race pace and walk 1 minute briskly. |
| Thu | Rest | Do as little activity as possible. Fridays are important rest days. In order for your muscles to grow stronger they need rest. |
| Fri | 4 miles (6.4 km) | Walk at your goal race pace. |

| Sat | 11 miles (17.6.4 km) | The most important part of your long duration walks is finishing the distance. Attempt to walk these at your half marathon goal race pace. This week's distance is closing in on a walk that might last over 3 hours. As the weeks continue, the distance required to walk becomes greater and greater. As the long duration walks continue to gradually increase, you might not be able to keep goal race pace. If this happens, don't sweat it, do the best you can and finish the distance. You're far better off to finish the distance at a slower pace than quit walking altogether because you're tired. |
|-----|------|------|
| Sun | Rest/CT 30 minutes | Rest or cross train. Since you're not planning on running the half marathon, you could easily cross train for thirty minutes in the activity of your choice. |
| **Notes** | | |
| | | |

- Get plenty of sleep the night before your long duration walk.
- Try to walk your long duration walk early in the morning.
- After each walk it's important to stretch out your muscles.
- If your long walks are taking up too much time, consider splitting up your walks into two different sessions possibly one in the morning and one at night.

# Marathon Training - Week 7

| | | |
|---|---|---|
| Mon | 4 miles (6.4 km) | Rest. Take it easy. Don't walk. If you need to exercise, I recommend a walk for no longer than 30 minutes. |
| Tue | CT 30 minutes | Cross train in an activity that complements your walking. Try not to walk since you're already walking during your normal training schedule. Try biking, yoga, weights, spin class, pump-it-up group class, etc. |
| Wed | 8 miles (12.8 km) | Perfect day to practice interval training. For example, walk at your goal race pace for 4 minutes and then speed up your pace for 1 minute. Repeat until you complete the distance for the day. You can change your intervals as well such as 3 minutes walking at goal race pace and 2 minutes walking briskly. Or you could walk 9 minutes goal race pace and walk 1 minute briskly. |
| Thu | Rest | Do as little activity as possible. Fridays are important rest days. In order for your muscles to grow stronger they need rest. |
| Fri | 4 miles (6.4 km) | Walk at your goal race pace. |

| Sat | 12 miles (19.2 km) | The most important part of your long duration walks is finishing the distance. Attempt to walk these at your half marathon goal race pace. This week's distance is closing in on a walk that might last over 3 hours. As the weeks continue, the distance required to walk becomes greater and greater. As the long duration walks continue to gradually increase, you might not be able to keep goal race pace. If this happens, don't sweat it, do the best you can and finish the distance. You're far better off to finish the distance at a slower pace than quit walking altogether because you're tired. |
| Sun | Rest/CT 30 minutes | Rest or cross train. Since you're not planning on running the half marathon, you could easily cross train for thirty minutes in the activity of your choice. |
| **Notes** | | |
| | | |

- Get plenty of sleep the night before your long duration walk.
- Try to walk your long duration walk early in the morning.
- After each walk it's important to stretch out your muscles.
- If your long walks are taking up too much time, consider splitting up your long distance walks into two different sessions possibly one in the morning and one at night.

# Marathon Training - Week 8

| Mon | 6 miles (9.6 km) | Rest. Take it easy. Don't walk. If you need to exercise, I recommend a walk for no longer than 30 minutes. |
|-----|------------------|-----------------------------------------------------------------------------------------------------------|
| Tue | CT 30 minutes | Cross train in an activity that complements your walking. Try not to walk since you're already walking during your normal training schedule. Try biking, yoga, weights, spin class, pump-it-up group class, etc. |
| Wed | 8 miles (12.8 km) | Perfect day to practice interval training. For example, walk at your goal race pace for 4 minutes and then speed up your pace for 1 minute. Repeat until you complete the distance for the day. You can change your intervals as well such as 3 minutes walking at goal race pace and 2 minutes walking briskly. Or you could walk 9 minutes goal race pace and walk 1 minute briskly. |
| Thu | Rest | Do as little activity as possible. Fridays are important rest days. In order for your muscles to grow stronger they need rest. |
| Fri | 4 miles (6.4 km) | Walk at your goal race pace. |

| Sat | 14 miles 22.4 km) | The most important part of your long duration walks is finishing the distance. Attempt to walk these at your half marathon goal race pace. This week's distance is closing in on a walk that might last over 3 hours. As the weeks continue, the distance required to walk becomes greater and greater. As the long duration walks continue to gradually increase, you might not be able to keep goal race pace. If this happens, don't sweat it, do the best you can and finish the distance. You're far better off to finish the distance at a slower pace than quit walking altogether because you're tired. |
|-----|-------------------|------------------------------------------------------------------------------------------------------------------------------------------------------------------------------------------------------------------------------------------------------------------------------------------------------------------------------------------------------------------------------------------------------------------------------------------------------------------------------------------------------------------------------------------------------------------------------------------------------------------------------------------|
| Sun | Rest/CT 30 minutes | Rest or cross train. Since you're not planning on running the half marathon, you could easily cross train for thirty minutes in the activity of your choice. |
| **Notes** | | |
| | | |

- Get plenty of sleep the night before your long duration walk.
- Try to walk your long duration walk early in the morning.
- After each walk it's important to stretch out your muscles.
- If your long walks are taking up too much time, consider splitting up your walks into two different sessions possibly one in the morning and one at night.

# Marathon Training - Week 9

| Mon | 6 miles (9.6 km) | Rest. Take it easy. Don't walk. If you need to exercise, I recommend a walk for no longer than 30 minutes. |
|---|---|---|
| Tue | CT 30 minutes | Cross train in an activity that complements your walking. Try not to walk since you're already walking during your normal training schedule. Try biking, yoga, weights, spin class, pump-it-up group class, etc. |
| Wed | 8 miles (12.8 km) | Perfect day to practice interval training. For example, walk at your goal race pace for 4 minutes and then speed up your pace for 1 minute. Repeat until you complete the distance for the day. You can change your intervals as well such as 3 minutes walking at goal race pace and 2 minutes walking briskly. Or you could walk 9 minutes goal race pace and walk 1 minute briskly. |
| Thu | Rest | Do as little activity as possible. Fridays are important rest days. In order for your muscles to grow stronger they need rest. |
| Fri | 4 miles (6.4 km) | Walk at your goal race pace. |

| Sat | 16 miles (25.6 km) | The most important part of your long duration walks is finishing the distance. Attempt to walk these at your half marathon goal race pace. This week's distance is closing in on a walk that might last over 3 hours. As the weeks continue, the distance required to walk becomes greater and greater. As the long duration walks continue to gradually increase, you might not be able to keep goal race pace. If this happens, don't sweat it, do the best you can and finish the distance. You're far better off to finish the distance at a slower pace than quit walking altogether because you're tired. |
| --- | --- | --- |
| Sun | Rest/CT 30 minutes | Rest or cross train. Since you're not planning on running the half marathon, you could easily cross train for thirty minutes in the activity of your choice. |
| **Notes** | | |
| | | |

- Get plenty of sleep the night before your long duration walk.
- Try to walk your long duration walk early in the morning.
- After each walk it's important to stretch out your muscles.
- If your long walks are taking up too much time, consider splitting up your walks into two different sessions possibly one in the morning and one at night.

# Marathon Training - Week 10

| Mon | 4 miles (6.4 km) | Rest. Take it easy. Don't walk. If you need to exercise, I recommend a walk for no longer than 30 minutes. |
|---|---|---|
| Tue | CT 30 minutes | Cross train in an activity that complements your walking. Try not to walk since you're already walking during your normal training schedule. Try biking, yoga, weights, spin class, pump-it-up group class, etc. |
| Wed | 4 miles (6.4 km) | Perfect day to practice interval training. For example, walk at your goal race pace for 4 minutes and then speed up your pace for 1 minute. Repeat until you complete the distance for the day. You can change your intervals as well such as 3 minutes walking at goal race pace and 2 minutes walking briskly. Or you could walk 9 minutes goal race pace and walk 1 minute briskly. |
| Thu | Rest | Do as little activity as possible. Fridays are important rest days. In order for your muscles to grow stronger they need rest. |
| Fri | 4 miles (6.4 km) | Walk at your goal race pace. |

| Sat | 13.1 miles (21 km)  Optional HM Race | The most important part of your long duration walks is finishing the distance. Attempt to walk these at your half marathon goal race pace. This week's distance is closing in on a walk that might last over 3 hours. As the weeks continue, the distance required to walk becomes greater and greater. As the long duration walks continue to gradually increase, you might not be able to keep goal race pace. If this happens, don't sweat it, do the best you can and finish the distance. You're far better off to finish the distance at a slower pace than quit walking altogether because you're tired. |
| Sun | Rest/CT 30 minutes | Rest or cross train. Since you're not planning on running the half marathon, you could easily cross train for thirty minutes in the activity of your choice. |
| **Notes** | | |
| | | |

- Get plenty of sleep the night before your long duration walk.
- Try to walk your long duration walk early in the morning.
- After each walk it's important to stretch out your muscles.
- If your long walks are taking up too much time, consider splitting up your walks into two different sessions possibly one in the morning and one at night.

# Marathon Training - Week 11

| | | |
|---|---|---|
| Mon | 6 miles (9.6 km) | Rest. Take it easy. Don't walk. If you need to exercise, I recommend a walk for no longer than 30 minutes. |
| Tue | CT 30 minutes | Cross train in an activity that complements your walking. Try not to walk since you're already walking during your normal training schedule. Try biking, yoga, weights, spin class, pump-it-up group class, etc. |
| Wed | 6 miles (9.6 km) | Perfect day to practice interval training. For example, walk at your goal race pace for 4 minutes and then speed up your pace for 1 minute. Repeat until you complete the distance for the day. You can change your intervals as well such as 3 minutes walking at goal race pace and 2 minutes walking briskly. Or you could walk 9 minutes goal race pace and walk 1 minute briskly. |
| Thu | Rest | Do as little activity as possible. Fridays are important rest days. In order for your muscles to grow stronger they need rest. |
| Fri | 4 miles (6.4 km) | Walk at your goal race pace. |

| Sat | 14 miles (22.4 km) | The most important part of your long duration walks is finishing the distance. Attempt to walk these at your half marathon goal race pace. This week's distance is closing in on a walk that might last over 3 hours. As the weeks continue, the distance required to walk becomes greater and greater. As the long duration walks continue to gradually increase, you might not be able to keep goal race pace. If this happens, don't sweat it, do the best you can and finish the distance. You're far better off to finish the distance at a slower pace than quit walking altogether because you're tired. |
|---|---|---|
| Sun | Rest/CT 30 minutes | Rest or cross train. Since you're not planning on running the half marathon, you could easily cross train for thirty minutes in the activity of your choice. |
| **Notes** | | |
| | | |

- Get plenty of sleep the night before your long duration walk.
- Try to walk your long duration walk early in the morning.
- After each walk it's important to stretch out your muscles.
- If your long walks are taking up too much time, consider splitting up your walks into two different sessions possibly one in the morning and one at night.

# Marathon Training - Week 12

| | | |
|---|---|---|
| Mon | 6 miles (9.6 km) | Rest. Take it easy. Don't walk. If you need to exercise, I recommend a walk for no longer than 30 minutes. |
| Tue | CT 30 minutes | Cross train in an activity that complements your walking. Try not to walk since you're already walking during your normal training schedule. Try biking, yoga, weights, spin class, pump-it-up group class, etc. |
| Wed | 8 miles (12.8 km) | Perfect day to practice interval training. For example, walk at your goal race pace for 4 minutes and then speed up your pace for 1 minute. Repeat until you complete the distance for the day. You can change your intervals as well such as 3 minutes walking at goal race pace and 2 minutes walking briskly. Or you could walk 9 minutes goal race pace and walk 1 minute briskly. |
| Thu | Rest | Do as little activity as possible. Fridays are important rest days. In order for your muscles to grow stronger they need rest. |
| Fri | 4 miles (6.4 km) | Walk at your goal race pace. |

| Sat | 16 miles (25.6 km) | The most important part of your long duration walks is finishing the distance. Attempt to walk these at your half marathon goal race pace. This week's distance is closing in on a walk that might last over 3 hours. As the weeks continue, the distance required to walk becomes greater and greater. As the long duration walks continue to gradually increase, you might not be able to keep goal race pace. If this happens, don't sweat it, do the best you can and finish the distance. You're far better off to finish the distance at a slower pace than quit walking altogether because you're tired. |
| Sun | Rest/CT 30 minutes | Rest or cross train. Since you're not planning on running the half marathon, you could easily cross train for thirty minutes in the activity of your choice. |
| **Notes** | | |
| | | |

- Get plenty of sleep the night before your long duration walk.
- Try to walk your long duration walk early in the morning.
- After each walk it's important to stretch out your muscles.
- If your long walks are taking up too much time, consider splitting up your walks into two different sessions possibly one in the morning and one at night.

# Marathon Training - Week 13

| Mon | 8 miles (12.8 km) | Rest. Take it easy. Don't walk. If you need to exercise, I recommend a walk for no longer than 30 minutes. |
|---|---|---|
| Tue | CT 30 minutes | Cross train in an activity that complements your walking. Try not to walk since you're already walking during your normal training schedule. Try biking, yoga, weights, spin class, pump-it-up group class, etc. |
| Wed | 10 miles (16 km) | Perfect day to practice interval training. For example, walk at your goal race pace for 4 minutes and then speed up your pace for 1 minute. Repeat until you complete the distance for the day. You can change your intervals as well such as 3 minutes walking at goal race pace and 2 minutes walking briskly. Or you could walk 9 minutes goal race pace and walk 1 minute briskly. |
| Thu | Rest | Do as little activity as possible. Fridays are important rest days. In order for your muscles to grow stronger they need rest. |
| Fri | 4 miles (6.4 km) | Walk at your goal race pace. |

| Sat | 18 miles (28.8 km) | The most important part of your long duration walks is finishing the distance. Attempt to walk these at your half marathon goal race pace. This week's distance is closing in on a walk that might last over 3 hours. As the weeks continue, the distance required to walk becomes greater and greater. As the long duration walks continue to gradually increase, you might not be able to keep goal race pace. If this happens, don't sweat it, do the best you can and finish the distance. You're far better off to finish the distance at a slower pace than quit walking altogether because you're tired. |
| --- | --- | --- |
| Sun | Rest/CT 30 minutes | Rest or cross train. Since you're not planning on running the half marathon, you could easily cross train for thirty minutes in the activity of your choice. |
| **Notes** | | |
| | | |

- Get plenty of sleep the night before your long duration walk.
- Try to walk your long duration walk early in the morning.
- After each walk it's important to stretch out your muscles.
- If your long walks are taking up too much time, consider splitting up your walks into two different sessions possibly one in the morning and one at night.

# Marathon Training - Week 14

| | | |
|---|---|---|
| Mon | 6 miles (9.6 km) | Rest. Take it easy. Don't walk. If you need to exercise, I recommend a walk for no longer than 30 minutes. |
| Tue | CT 30 minutes | Cross train in an activity that complements your walking. Try not to walk since you're already walking during your normal training schedule. Try biking, yoga, weights, spin class, pump-it-up group class, etc. |
| Wed | 10 miles (16 km) | Perfect day to practice interval training. For example, walk at your goal race pace for 4 minutes and then speed up your pace for 1 minute. Repeat until you complete the distance for the day. You can change your intervals as well such as 3 minutes walking at goal race pace and 2 minutes walking briskly. Or you could walk 9 minutes goal race pace and walk 1 minute briskly. |
| Thu | Rest | Do as little activity as possible. Fridays are important rest days. In order for your muscles to grow stronger they need rest. |
| Fri | 4 miles (6.4 km) | Walk at your goal race pace. |

| | | |
|---|---|---|
| Sat | 20 miles (32 km) | The most important part of your long duration walks is finishing the distance. Attempt to walk these at your half marathon goal race pace. This week's distance is closing in on a walk that might last over 3 hours. As the weeks continue, the distance required to walk becomes greater and greater. As the long duration walks continue to gradually increase, you might not be able to keep goal race pace. If this happens, don't sweat it, do the best you can and finish the distance. You're far better off to finish the distance at a slower pace than quit walking altogether because you're tired. |
| Sun | Rest/CT 30 minutes | Rest or cross train. Since you're not planning on running the half marathon, you could easily cross train for thirty minutes in the activity of your choice. |
| **Notes** | | |
| | | |

- Get plenty of sleep the night before your long duration walk.
- Try to walk your long duration walk early in the morning.
- After each walk it's important to stretch out your muscles.
- If your long walks are taking up too much time, consider splitting up your walks into two different sessions possibly one in the morning and one at night.

# Marathon Training - Week 15

| Mon | 8 miles (12.8 km) | Rest. Take it easy. Don't walk. If you need to exercise, I recommend a walk for no longer than 30 minutes. |
|---|---|---|
| Tue | CT 30 minutes | Cross train in an activity that complements your walking. Try not to walk since you're already walking during your normal training schedule. Try biking, yoga, weights, spin class, pump-it-up group class, etc. |
| Wed | 10 miles (16 km) | Perfect day to practice interval training. For example, walk at your goal race pace for 4 minutes and then speed up your pace for 1 minute. Repeat until you complete the distance for the day. You can change your intervals as well such as 3 minutes walking at goal race pace and 2 minutes walking briskly. Or you could walk 9 minutes goal race pace and walk 1 minute briskly. |
| Thu | Rest | Do as little activity as possible. Fridays are important rest days. In order for your muscles to grow stronger they need rest. |
| Fri | 4 miles (6.4 km) | Walk at your goal race pace. |

| Sat | 22 miles (35.2 km) | The most important part of your long duration walks is finishing the distance. Attempt to walk these at your half marathon goal race pace. This week's distance is closing in on a walk that might last over 3 hours. As the weeks continue, the distance required to walk becomes greater and greater. As the long duration walks continue to gradually increase, you might not be able to keep goal race pace. If this happens, don't sweat it, do the best you can and finish the distance. You're far better off to finish the distance at a slower pace than quit walking altogether because you're tired. |
|-----|-----|-----|
| Sun | Rest/CT 30 minutes | Rest or cross train. Since you're not planning on running the half marathon, you could easily cross train for thirty minutes in the activity of your choice. |
| **Notes** | | |
|  | | |

- Get plenty of sleep the night before your long duration walk.
- Try to walk your long duration walk early in the morning.
- After each walk it's important to stretch out your muscles.
- If your long walks are taking up too much time, consider splitting up your walks into two different sessions possibly one in the morning and one at night.

# Marathon Training - Week 16

| Mon | 6 miles (9.6 km) | Rest. Take it easy. Don't walk. If you need to exercise, I recommend a walk for no longer than 30 minutes. |
|---|---|---|
| Tue | CT 30 minutes | Cross train in an activity that complements your walking. Try not to walk since you're already walking during your normal training schedule. Try biking, yoga, weights, spin class, pump-it-up group class, etc. |
| Wed | 8 miles (12.8 km) | Perfect day to practice interval training. For example, walk at your goal race pace for 4 minutes and then speed up your pace for 1 minute. Repeat until you complete the distance for the day. You can change your intervals as well such as 3 minutes walking at goal race pace and 2 minutes walking briskly. Or you could walk 9 minutes goal race pace and walk 1 minute briskly. |
| Thu | Rest | Do as little activity as possible. Fridays are important rest days. In order for your muscles to grow stronger they need rest. |
| Fri | 4 miles (6.4 km) | Walk at your goal race pace. |

| Sat | 18 miles (28.8 km) | The most important part of your long duration walks is finishing the distance. Attempt to walk these at your half marathon goal race pace. This week's distance is closing in on a walk that might last over 3 hours. As the weeks continue, the distance required to walk becomes greater and greater. As the long duration walks continue to gradually increase, you might not be able to keep goal race pace. If this happens, don't sweat it, do the best you can and finish the distance. You're far better off to finish the distance at a slower pace than quit walking altogether because you're tired. |
| --- | --- | --- |
| Sun | Rest/CT 30 minutes | Rest or cross train. Since you're not planning on running the half marathon, you could easily cross train for thirty minutes in the activity of your choice. |
| **Notes** | | |
| | | |

- Get plenty of sleep the night before your long duration walk.
- Try to walk your long duration walk early in the morning.
- After each walk it's important to stretch out your muscles.
- If your long walks are taking up too much time, consider splitting up your walks into two different sessions possibly one in the morning and one at night.

# Marathon Training - Week 17

| Mon | 4 miles (6.4 km) | Rest. Take it easy. Don't walk. If you need to exercise, I recommend a walk for no longer than 30 minutes. |
|---|---|---|
| Tue | CT 30 minutes | Cross train in an activity that complements your walking. Try not to walk since you're already walking during your normal training schedule. Try biking, yoga, weights, spin class, pump-it-up group class, etc. |
| Wed | 6 miles (9.6 km) | Perfect day to practice interval training. For example, walk at your goal race pace for 4 minutes and then speed up your pace for 1 minute. Repeat until you complete the distance for the day. You can change your intervals as well such as 3 minutes walking at goal race pace and 2 minutes walking briskly. Or you could walk 9 minutes goal race pace and walk 1 minute briskly. |
| Thu | Rest | Do as little activity as possible. Fridays are important rest days. In order for your muscles to grow stronger they need rest. |
| Fri | 4 miles (6.4 km) | Walk at your goal race pace. |

| Sat | 12 miles (19.2 km) | The most important part of your long duration walks is finishing the distance. Attempt to walk these at your half marathon goal race pace. This week's distance is closing in on a walk that might last over 3 hours. As the weeks continue, the distance required to walk becomes greater and greater. As the long duration walks continue to gradually increase, you might not be able to keep goal race pace. If this happens, don't sweat it, do the best you can and finish the distance. You're far better off to finish the distance at a slower pace than quit walking altogether because you're tired. |
| Sun | Rest/CT 30 minutes | Rest or cross train. Since you're not planning on running the half marathon, you could easily cross train for thirty minutes in the activity of your choice. |
| **Notes** | | |
| | | |

- Get plenty of sleep the night before your long duration walk.
- Try to walk your long duration walk early in the morning.
- After each walk it's important to stretch out your muscles.
- If your long walks are taking up too much time, consider splitting up your walks into two different sessions possibly one in the morning and one at night.

# Marathon Training - Week 18

| | | |
|---|---|---|
| Mon | 4 miles (6.4 km) | Walk at your goal race pace. |
| Tue | CT 30 minutes | Cross train in an activity that complements your walking. Try not to walk since you're already walking during your normal training schedule. Try biking, yoga, weights, spin class, pump-it-up group class, etc. |
| Wed | 6 miles (9.6 km) | Walk at your goal race pace. |
| Thu | Rest | Do as little activity as possible. Fridays are important rest days. In order for your muscles to grow stronger they need rest. |
| Fri | 4 miles (6.4 km) | Walk at your goal race pace. |
| Sat | 26.2 miles (42 km) | RACE DAY! |
| Sun | Rest | Rest and celebrate your victory! |

| **Notes** |
| --- |
| |

- Get plenty of sleep the night before your long duration walk.
- Try to walk your long duration walk early in the morning.
- After each walk it's important to stretch out your muscles.
- If your long walks are taking up too much time, consider splitting up your walks into two different sessions possibly one in the morning and one at night.
- This week your body needs as much rest as possible.

# Part V - Race Day

# Two Days Before the Race

You will want to eat carbohydrates with every meal. Pasta, rice, and bread are all good sources of carbohydrates to store as glycogen for your race. The week of your race is not the time to overeat. Substitute fruits or vegetables for a serving of carbohydrates. Get plenty of rest. You will gain weight the week leading up to your race. You should lose some weight during your walk. The night which is two nights before your race is going to be your best chance to get a full night of sleep.

# Night Before the Race

A lot of people will find it difficult to get enough sleep the night before your first half marathon. Some runners will walk a few light miles the day before the race. Lay out your race gear so that it will be ready in the morning — just like you've done on each long run training session—which includes your clothing, tech gear, waters, gels, hydration packs, water bottles, running shoes, and socks. If you picked up your race packet early, go ahead and pin the racing number on your shirt or shorts. Do not drink alcohol. If you do drink alcohol, limit yourself to a few drinks. Your body will thank you on race day.

# Race Day

The day has finally arrived. Wake up a couple of hours early before the race start time. (Yeah, I know it's early). Eat a small meal as soon as you wake up. This meal should have some carbohydrates, such as a bagel or toast with peanut butter, maybe a few eggs, and water. Avoid high fiber content food. This meal should be identical to the meals you ate before all your successful long duration walks. You don't want to change up your routine on race day. I have heard too many stories of people getting sick during a race because they consumed "extra" gels or changed out an energy replacement for something else offered at the race. Stick to your training plan. Drink a cup or two of coffee and drink about 12 oz of water before the race. Continue to sip on water leading up to the race. Remember you don't want a sloshing stomach, so don't over drink. Your body should be hydrated if you began your hydration two days before race day and cut out most alcoholic beverages.

When people begin to line up for the race, you need to pick the correct starting location in the herd. At most large marathons you will be corralled into finish times to help separate and break up the flow of traffic. If there are no corrals and this is your first half marathon, do not line up at the front of the starting line unless you are going to run the half marathon in 1 hour and 30 minutes. The announcer will state this over and over up until race time. You could easily get stampeded if you attempt to do this or you could hurt someone else. The slowest paced walkers need to be in the back of the queue. The average paced runners should be in the middle of the herd. I have, on many races, thought I was in the correct location somewhere in the middle, and I was wrong. I had to pass many, many people performing slot type racing just to get out of the muck of people. If you are running the race, you need to be in the front of the pack. Roughly between the first 20% and 60% of the racers. The racers at the tail end are planning on walking at a much slower pace. If you need to slow down your pace, then you need to move to the right of the course.

Your blood is pumping, the caffeine is kicking, and the announcer is counting down the last ten seconds before race time. You hear the gun announce the start of the race and you start walking way faster than you trained. You reach the 2nd mile still moving at an above average training pace time. You reach the third mile, and you must slow down because you are out of breath from nearly sprinting the last three miles. Now your overall total chip time will be much worse than it had been during training. Take it easy out of the gate. Conserve your energy. Steady and even pacing just like your long-distance training will get you through the race. You will notice that your pace per mile will be faster than your training pace. The excitement, adrenaline and competitive aspects of the race naturally add to the energy surging through your body. So, take it slow at first and walk at the pace you've trained at over the last 12 to 18 weeks.

# Post-Race

Your body is exhausted, and you might even be a little emotional right now, hanging on to your new, shiny medal, but don't sit down when you cross the finish line. At a bare minimum keep walking for another 10 to 20 minutes. If your body feels like it, jog at a light pace for another 10 minutes. Grab something to drink with electrolytes if possible. You need to eat something within at least one hour after your race, to help replenish your body with nutrients and liquids.

If you're up for it, you can drink a beer or two. Drink plenty of water and keep yourself hydrated over the next couple of days. Sometimes a recovery walk the next day will help stretch out some of your sore leg muscles. Your recovery walk should be at a light pace and not last more than thirty minutes.

How long do you have to wait before you start training again? This depends on your age, your body, your recovery time, etc. If your half-marathon was on the way to a full marathon, then you should be ready to start your next long session within five days. You might need to adjust your other walks for the upcoming week due to the exertion you put forth in the half marathon race. If this is the end of the line for your racing for a while, just take it easy for at least a week. If you get antsy, then go ahead and start walking again when your body feels like it. Just remember that your body will be tired for several days after your half marathon or marathon. Listen to your body. For example, if you are walking 4 miles just 4 days after your half marathon or marathon and you start to get winded, that's a sign that your body is still exhausted.

Wait one week before you walk more than 5 miles in one running session. Wait two weeks before you walk more than 9 miles in one training session.

# Action Steps

Two days before the race:
- You should be tapering now.
- Start hydrating - no alcohol.
- Replace some of your food with dense carb food such as pasta and whole grain breads.
- Get at least 7 hours of sleep.

One day before the race:
- Get all your gear laid out, including clothes, gels, water, phone, Garmins, and Fitbits.
- Attach your bib number to your clothes.
- Know what route you are going to take to the race.
- Keep hydrating.
- Your last dinner before the race, do not eat a big meal.
- Get at least 7 hours of sleep (might be hard to do this because of anxiety).
- If you are getting edgy, go for a mile or two walk.

Race day:
- Wake up at least two hours before your race.
- Eat as soon as you get up. Oatmeal, energy bars, and a banana are great sources of food.
- This meal should be the same as your long-distance training sessions.
- Drink some caffeine 1-2 hours before the race.
- Keep sipping water up until race time.
- Don't consume too much water. If your stomach is sloshing around, you drank too much.
- Arrive at the race a little early if possible, just in case of traffic.

- If you plan on taking a gel before the race, take it about 5-15 minutes before the race.

The Race:
- Don't burst out of the starting line like lightning.
- Race like you trained and you will finish the race.
- Gels taken during the race need to be taken with water for proper assimilation.
- If you are taking energy gels during the race, you won't need to drink sport drinks. Your gels will have enough electrolytes in them.
- Remember you don't have to go full steam the entire race. Slow down to a brisk walk at the water/aid stations for 1/10 mile or 2 minutes then speed back up.

Post-Race:
- Don't stop moving at the finish line.
- Keep walking for 10 to 20 minutes after the race.
- Grab a sports drink and some food such as a banana, yogurt, or bread.
- Pose for pictures and enjoy your new, shiny medal.
- Stretch your muscles accordingly.

# Conclusion

# Congratulations

Pat yourself on the back if you've completed your first marathon or marathon. No matter how long it took you to finish your race, remember that you did something awesome today while other people sat on the couch. Congratulations!

# I NEED YOUR HELP

Thanks for reading! If you've enjoyed this book, please leave me a 5-star gleaming review by simply stating one or two sentences describing what you liked best about the book. Other shoppers on Amazon rely on ratings so that it can save them valuable time when shopping for new books. I take the time to read each review. Your help and support are very much appreciated.

If you've just finished a race and you want someone to tell, send me an email. I would be delighted to hear from you.

**Follow me:**

Facebook: facebook.com/BeginnerToFinisher
SoundCloud: Audiobooks
Twitter:@BeginR2FinishR
Instagram:Beginnr2Finishr
Tumblr:Tumblr
Amazon: Amazon Author Page
Amazon Storefront: Beginner to Finisher
Website: www.halfmarathonforbeginners.com
Email: scottmorton@halfmarathonforbeginners.com

# What's Next?

If you want to slowly transition into running, you can check out my running series, *Beginner to Finisher*. This series takes you through the ultra-basics of running all the way up to the half marathon (marathon book coming soon). If you have no desire to run, then continue seeking walker friendly half marathons and marathons and try to beat a personal best.

Click here to check out the series

If you're still unsure of where to start or have other questions regarding running for beginners, please read the first book in the series, Beginner to Finisher Book 1:

**CLICK BELOW ON LINK:**
*Why New Runners Fail: 26 Ultimate Tips You Should Know Before You Start Running!*

# About the Author

I played sports throughout my youth and even into my adult years. I ran my first 5k at the age of 37 in March of 2008 without any training at all. I finished third place, although my leg muscles felt like I deserved first place. My legs were sore for six days after the race. My next 5k attempt was in 2015 at the age of 42 in my local hometown. I had no intention of placing at all. I ended up running worse than my first 5k by almost two minutes. I placed second with no training at all. I thought I would have learned a lesson by now - nope.

In May 2016, I was flying to Las Vegas for our yearly guys' trip. I was reading a *Sky Mall* magazine, and I came across an article called "Top 100 things to do in Las Vegas." Number eight on the list was run a race through the streets of Las Vegas. During the race, the city blocks off sections of the strip. I was hooked. They offered a 5k, 10k, half marathon and marathon. I liked walking a lot; in fact, one of my favorite things to do in Las Vegas was to see how many steps I could get in a day (my record to date is 42,000). The Rock-and-Roll Half Marathon/Marathon would be taking place in November 2016. I scoured the Internet for any information related to training for a half marathon.

My wife asked me, "Why in the world do you want to run a half marathon?" I told her because I was physically able to. She said, "You just want to put one of those 13.1 stickers on the back of your car." But truthfully the real reason was much deeper than that. Whenever I catch a fresh dump of powder on my snowboard, there is no other experience like it. I feel like a kid again, and I feel alive. The real reason I wanted to run was because I wanted to feel the accomplishment, feel the pain and feel the glory of crossing the finish line all the while feeling alive. Running allows me to unleash that competitive kid inside me who yearns to feel alive.

In Nov 2018, Scott became an RRCA certified coach, and to date has completed 10 half marathons and 1 full marathon.

Printed in Great Britain
by Amazon

58293840R00076